JUICING FOR CANCER

15+ Nourishing Recipes to boost your immunity and promote wellness

Marybeth Watson

CHAPTER 6: RECIPES FOR JUICES THAT FIGHT CANCER

CHAPTER 7: SMOOTHIES FOR CANCER PATIENTS

CHAPTER 8: NUTRITIOUS SNACKS FOR CANCER PATIENTS

CONCLUSION

Introduction

Welcome to "Juicing for Cancer Recipes Book: 15+ Nourishing Recipes to Boost Your Immunity and Promote Wellness". If you or someone you love has been affected by cancer, you know how overwhelming the journey can be. The physical and emotional tolls of the disease and its treatments can be challenging to manage, and it's essential to take care of your body and mind during this time.

One way to support your health and well-being is through juicing. Juicing provides an easy and delicious way to consume a wide variety of fruits, vegetables, and herbs, which are rich in nutrients that can help boost your immune system, reduce inflammation, and support your body's natural detoxification processes.

In this book, you'll find over 15 juicing recipes that are specifically designed for cancer patients and those looking to prevent cancer. Each recipe includes a detailed list of ingredients and instructions, as well as information on the health benefits of the key ingredients.

We've also included tips on how to safely and effectively juice, how to store your juices for optimal freshness, and how to choose the best produce for your needs.

We hope this book will inspire you to incorporate juicing into your daily routine and help you discover the healing power of fruits, vegetables, and herbs. Remember, every small step you take towards better health is a step in the right direction. Let's get juicing!

Chapter 1: Understanding Cancer and its Impact on the Body

Cancer is a complex and multifactorial disease that affects millions of people worldwide. It is characterized by the abnormal growth and spread of cells in the body, which can lead to a range of symptoms and complications. In this chapter, we will explore the meaning of cancer, How Cancer Affects the Body and the Common Types of Cancer.

What is Cancer?

Cancer is a disease characterized by the uncontrolled growth and spread of abnormal cells in the body. These abnormal cells are known as cancer cells and can form tumors, invade surrounding tissue, and even spread to other parts of the body. Cancer can occur in any part of the body and can affect any tissue or organ.

Cancer develops when the normal control mechanisms in the body stop working. Old cells do not die and instead continue to grow and divide, creating more and more abnormal cells. These abnormal cells can form a mass of tissue called a tumor. Tumors can be benign, meaning they are not cancerous and do not spread to other parts of the body, or they can be malignant, which means they are cancerous and can spread to other parts of the body.

Cancer cells are different from normal cells in several ways. For example, cancer cells can divide and grow more quickly than normal cells. They can also ignore signals that tell them to stop dividing or die. Cancer cells can even produce their own blood supply to help them grow and spread.

How Cancer Affects the Body

Cancer can affect any part of the body, from the skin to the brain. Depending on the type and stage of cancer, it can affect tissues and organs in different ways.

For example, lung cancer can affect the lungs, making it difficult to breathe and causing coughing and chest pain. Breast cancer can affect the breasts, causing lumps, nipple discharge, and changes in the skin. Prostate cancer can affect the prostate gland, causing difficulty urinating and sexual dysfunction.

As cancer progresses, it can spread to nearby tissues and organs, causing further damage and complications. For example, advanced lung cancer can spread to the bones, causing pain and fractures, or to the brain, causing headaches, seizures, and other neurological symptoms.

Cancer is not just a physical disease, but it can also have a significant impact on a patient's mental health. The diagnosis of cancer can be emotionally devastating and can trigger a range of psychological symptoms, including anxiety, depression, and fear.

Anxiety is a common emotional response to cancer, and it can cause physical symptoms such as racing heart, sweating, and shortness of breath. Anxiety can also lead to sleep disturbances, irritability, and difficulty concentrating, which can further impact a patient's quality of life.

Depression is another common mental health issue that can occur in cancer patients. It can cause persistent feelings of sadness, hopelessness, and worthlessness, leading to a loss of interest in activities that once brought pleasure. Depression can also cause physical symptoms such as fatigue, changes in appetite, and sleep disturbances.

In conclusion, cancer can have a significant impact on a patient's mental health, and it is essential to address both physical and psychological symptoms of cancer. Cancer patients should receive comprehensive care that includes not only treatment for their physical symptoms but also support for their mental health and well-being. Psychotherapy, support groups, and medications can all be effective in addressing mental health issues in cancer patients and improving their quality of life.

Common Types of Cancer

Breast Cancer

Breast cancer is the most common cancer in women worldwide, with more than 2 million new cases diagnosed every year. It occurs when cells in the breast tissue begin to grow and divide uncontrollably, forming a lump or mass. The risk of breast cancer increases with age, family history, and certain genetic mutations. Symptoms may include a lump or thickening in the breast, nipple discharge or inversion, and changes in breast shape or size. Early detection through mammograms and self-exams can improve the chances of successful treatment. Treatment options may include surgery, radiation therapy, chemotherapy, hormone therapy, and targeted therapy.

Lung Cancer

Lung cancer is the second most common cancer in both men and women, accounting for around 2 million new cases each year. It occurs when cells in the lungs grow and divide uncontrollably, forming a tumor that can spread to other parts of the body. The primary cause of lung cancer is tobacco smoke, which accounts for around 80% of all cases. Symptoms may include a persistent cough, chest pain, shortness of breath, and coughing up blood. Treatment options may include surgery, radiation therapy, chemotherapy, targeted therapy, and immunotherapy.

Prostate Cancer

Prostate cancer is the most common cancer in men, with more than 1 million new cases diagnosed worldwide each year. It occurs when cells in the prostate gland begin to grow and divide uncontrollably, forming a tumor. The risk of prostate cancer increases with age, family history, and certain genetic mutations. Symptoms may include difficulty urinating, frequent urination, blood in the urine, and pain or discomfort during ejaculation. Treatment options may include surgery, radiation therapy, hormone therapy, and chemotherapy.

Skin Cancer

Skin cancer is the most common type of cancer in the United States, with more than 5 million cases diagnosed each year. It occurs when cells in the skin begin to grow and divide uncontrollably, forming a tumor. The primary risk factor for skin cancer is exposure to ultraviolet (UV) radiation from the sun or tanning beds. Symptoms may include changes in the size, shape, or color of a mole or other skin lesion. Treatment options may include surgery, radiation therapy, chemotherapy, targeted therapy, and immunotherapy.

Bladder Cancer

Bladder cancer is the fourth most common cancer in men and the ninth most common cancer in women, with more than 500,000 new cases diagnosed each year. It occurs when cells in the lining of the bladder begin to grow and divide uncontrollably, forming a tumor. The primary risk factors for bladder cancer include smoking, exposure to certain chemicals, and chronic bladder infections. Symptoms may include blood in the urine, pain or discomfort during urination, and frequent urination. Treatment options may include surgery, radiation therapy, chemotherapy, and immunotherapy.

Leukemia

Leukemia is a type of cancer that affects the blood and bone marrow, with more than 400,000 new cases diagnosed worldwide each year. It occurs when abnormal white blood cells are produced in the bone marrow, which can interfere with the production of normal blood cells. The primary risk factors for leukemia include exposure to radiation or certain chemicals, certain genetic conditions, and a weakened immune system. Symptoms may include fatigue, weakness, recurrent infections, easy bruising or bleeding, and swollen lymph nodes. Treatment options may include chemotherapy, radiation therapy, stem cell transplantation, and targeted therapy.

Ovarian Cancer

Ovarian cancer is a type of cancer that affects the ovaries, with more than 295,000 new cases diagnosed worldwide each year. It occurs when cells in the ovaries begin to grow and divide uncontrollably, forming a tumor. The primary risk factors for ovarian cancer include age, family history, certain genetic mutations, and a history of infertility or hormone therapy. Symptoms may include bloating, pelvic pain or pressure, abdominal swelling, and changes in bowel or bladder habits. Treatment options may include surgery, chemotherapy, and targeted therapy.

Pancreatic Cancer

Pancreatic cancer is a type of cancer that affects the pancreas, with more than 450,000 new cases diagnosed worldwide each year. It occurs when cells in the pancreas begin to grow and divide uncontrollably, forming a tumor. The primary risk factors for pancreatic cancer include age, smoking, obesity, and a family history of the disease. Symptoms may include abdominal pain or discomfort, jaundice, weight loss, and nausea or vomiting. Treatment options may include surgery, radiation therapy, chemotherapy, targeted therapy, and immunotherapy.

Chapter 2: The Benefits of Juicing for Cancer Patients

Cancer is a devastating disease that affects millions of people every year. While traditional medical treatments like chemotherapy and radiation can be effective, they often have significant side effects that can make it difficult for patients to maintain their quality of life. As such, many cancer patients are turning to alternative therapies, including juicing, to help alleviate symptoms and support their overall health and wellness.

Juicing has become an increasingly popular way of consuming fruits and vegetables. While it has long been touted as a health trend, juicing is also a valuable tool for cancer patients. Cancer treatments, such as chemotherapy and radiation, can be hard on the body, causing fatigue, nausea, and a weakened immune system. Juicing provides an easy and convenient way to get the nutrients that the body needs to maintain strength and energy, while supporting the immune system. In this chapter, we will explore ways on how juicing can help prevent Cancer, how juicing can help fight cancer and the Nutritional benefits of juicing.

How Juicing Can Help Prevent Cancer

Cancer is a debilitating disease that affects millions of people worldwide. While there is no cure for cancer, there are several things that people can do to reduce their risk of developing this disease. One of these things is incorporating juicing into their diet. Juicing is an excellent way to get a concentrated dose of vitamins, minerals, and antioxidants that can help prevent cancer.

There is a growing body of research suggesting that juicing can help prevent cancer. The following are some of the ways in which juicing can help:

Juicing increases nutrient intake

Juicing allows you to consume a large number of fruits and vegetables in a short amount of time. This means that you can get a concentrated dose of vitamins, minerals, and antioxidants that can help prevent cancer.

Some of the best fruits and vegetables for cancer prevention include:

Leafy greens: Kale, spinach, and collard greens are all rich in antioxidants and can help prevent cancer.

Cruciferous vegetables: Broccoli, cauliflower, and cabbage contain compounds that have been shown to prevent cancer.

Berries: Blueberries, raspberries, and strawberries are all rich in antioxidants and can help prevent cancer.

Citrus fruits: Oranges, lemons, and limes contain vitamin C, a powerful antioxidant that can help prevent cancer.

Juicing reduces inflammation

Inflammation is a natural response to injury or infection, but chronic inflammation can lead to cancer. Some of the compounds found in fruits and vegetables have anti-inflammatory properties that can help reduce the risk of cancer. Juicing can help reduce inflammation by providing a concentrated dose of these compounds.

Juicing promotes detoxification

Toxins can accumulate in our bodies and lead to cancer. Juicing can help promote detoxification by providing a concentrated dose of nutrients that support liver function. The liver is responsible for filtering toxins from the body, and certain fruits and vegetables can help support its function.

Juicing can improve immune function

A strong immune system is essential for preventing cancer. Juicing can help improve immune function by providing a concentrated dose of nutrients that support immune function. Some of the best fruits and vegetables for immune function include:

Citrus fruits: Oranges, lemons, and limes contain vitamin C, which is essential for immune function.

Garlic: Garlic contains compounds that have been shown to boost immune function.

Ginger: Ginger contains compounds that have anti-inflammatory and immune-boosting properties.

Leafy greens: Leafy greens are rich in vitamins and minerals that are essential for immune function.

Juicing can help maintain a healthy weight

Obesity is a risk factor for several types of cancer. Juicing can help maintain a healthy weight by providing a concentrated dose of nutrients without adding extra calories. Additionally, fruits and vegetables are high in fiber, which can help keep you feeling full and prevent overeating.

Specific Fruits and Vegetables for Cancer Prevention
While all fruits and vegetables can help prevent cancer, some are particularly effective. The following are some of the best fruits and vegetables for cancer prevention:

Cruciferous Vegetables

Cruciferous vegetables like broccoli, cauliflower, and cabbage are rich in compounds called glucosinolates. These compounds have been shown to have cancer-preventive properties. When glucosinolates are broken down, they form compounds like indoles and isothiocyanates, which have been shown to help prevent cancer. Juicing these vegetables can provide a concentrated dose of these cancer-fighting compounds.

Berries

Berries like blueberries, raspberries, and strawberries are rich in antioxidants called anthocyanins. These compounds have been shown to have anti-cancer properties. They can help prevent cancer by reducing inflammation and protecting cells from damage caused by free radicals. Juicing these fruits can provide a concentrated dose of these cancer-fighting antioxidants.

Leafy Greens

Leafy greens like kale, spinach, and collard greens are rich in antioxidants like carotenoids and flavonoids. These compounds have been shown to have anti-cancer properties. They can help prevent cancer by reducing inflammation and protecting cells from damage caused by free radicals. Juicing these vegetables can provide a concentrated dose of these cancer-fighting antioxidants.

Citrus Fruits

Citrus fruits like oranges, lemons, and limes are rich in vitamin C, a powerful antioxidant that can help prevent cancer. Vitamin C has been shown to have anti-cancer properties by reducing inflammation and protecting cells from damage caused by free radicals. Juicing these fruits can provide a concentrated dose of vitamin C, making it easier to get the recommended daily intake.

Turmeric

Turmeric is a spice that has been used for centuries in traditional medicine. It contains a compound called curcumin, which has been shown to have anti-cancer properties. Curcumin has been shown to help prevent cancer by reducing inflammation and inhibiting the growth of cancer cells. Juicing turmeric can provide a concentrated dose of curcumin, making it easier to get the recommended daily intake.

Juicing is an excellent way to get a concentrated dose of vitamins, minerals, and antioxidants that can help prevent cancer. By incorporating juicing into your diet, you can increase your nutrient intake, reduce inflammation, promote detoxification, improve immune function, and maintain a healthy weight. Additionally, specific fruits and vegetables like cruciferous vegetables, berries, leafy greens, citrus fruits, and turmeric have been shown to have anti-cancer properties. Juicing these foods can provide a concentrated dose of cancer-fighting compounds, making it easier to get the recommended daily intake. While juicing is not a cure for cancer, it can be a powerful tool in the prevention of this devastating disease.

How Juicing Can Help Fight Cancer

Juicing is a powerful tool in fighting cancer due to its ability to provide the body with essential nutrients and antioxidants. The nutrients found in fruits and vegetables play a vital role in the body's ability to fight cancer by providing the necessary vitamins and minerals that help the body's immune system function optimally.

A healthy digestive system is crucial in the fight against cancer. Juicing can help to improve digestion by providing the body with digestive enzymes found in fruits and vegetables. These enzymes help to break down food, making it easier for the body to absorb nutrients. When the body is able to absorb nutrients more efficiently, it is better equipped to fight cancer.

Chapter 3: The Basics of Juicing

Juicing is the process of extracting juice from fruits and vegetables. It has become increasingly popular over the years as people look for ways to incorporate more nutrients into their diets. Juicing offers a simple and convenient way to consume a large amount of vitamins, minerals, and antioxidants in a single glass. In this chapter, we'll cover the basics of juicing, which includes The types of Juicers, Choosing the Right Ingredients, Preparing Your Produce and Tips for Juicing.

Types of Juicers

Juicing is an excellent way to enjoy a variety of healthy, delicious fruits and vegetables. With the help of a juicer, you can extract the maximum amount of juice from your produce, and enjoy a refreshing and nutritious drink. Juicers come in many different types, each with their own strengths and weaknesses. In this section, we will explore the different types of juicers available, how they work, and the benefits and drawbacks of each.

Centrifugal Juicers:

Centrifugal juicers are the most common type of juicer and are widely available in most stores. They work by spinning the produce at high speeds and then using centrifugal force to separate the juice from the pulp. These juicers are easy to use and can juice a variety of fruits and vegetables quickly. However, they are not as efficient as other types of juicers and can produce a less nutritious juice.

Pros:

- Fast and easy to use
- Can juice most fruits and vegetables
- Affordable

Cons:

- Not as efficient as other juicers
- Can produce a less nutritious juice
- Loud and can create a lot of foam

Masticating Juicers:

Masticating juicers, also known as slow juicers or cold-press juicers, work by crushing the produce and then pressing it to extract the juice. These juicers operate at a slower speed than centrifugal juicers, which results in a more nutrient-dense juice. They are also more versatile and can juice a wider variety of fruits and vegetables, including leafy greens and wheatgrass.

Pros:

- Produce a more nutrient-dense juice
- Can juice a wider variety of fruits and vegetables
- Quieter than centrifugal juicers

Cons:

- Slower than centrifugal juicers
- More expensive than centrifugal juicers
- Can be more difficult to clean

Twin Gear Juicers:

Twin gear juicers, also known as triturating juicers, use two gears that rotate in opposite directions to crush and press the produce. This type of juicer is even more efficient than masticating juicers, producing an even more nutrient-dense juice. They are also capable of juicing a wider variety of produce, including hard vegetables and fruits like carrots and apples.

Pros:

- Produce an even more nutrient-dense juice than masticating juicers
- Can juice a wider variety of fruits and vegetables
- Quiet operation

Cons:

- Expensive
- Can be more difficult to clean
- Slower than centrifugal and masticating juicers

Hydraulic Press Juicers:

Hydraulic press juicers are the most advanced type of juicer and are often used in commercial settings. They work by first crushing the produce and then pressing it through a hydraulic press to extract the juice. This type of juicer produces the most nutrient-dense juice, but it is also the most expensive and least practical for home use.

Pros:

- Produces the most nutrient-dense juice
- Ideal for commercial use

Cons:

- Very expensive
- Not practical for home use
- Requires a lot of space

Citrus Juicers:

Citrus juicers are designed specifically for juicing citrus fruits like oranges, lemons, and limes. They come in both manual and electric models and can be very affordable. These juicers are easy to use and can produce a lot of juice quickly. They are also easy to clean and maintain.

Pros:

- Affordable

- Easy to use

- Produce a lot of juice quickly

Cons:

- Only suitable for juicing citrus fruits

- Limited versatility

Auger Juicers:

Auger juicers, also known as single gear juicers, work by using a slowly rotating auger to crush the produce and extract the juice. This type of juicer operates at a slower speed than centrifugal juicers, which results in a more nutrient-dense juice. They are also more efficient than centrifugal juicers and can juice a wider variety of produce, including leafy greens and wheatgrass.

Pros:

- Produce a more nutrient-dense juice than centrifugal juicers
- Can juice a wider variety of fruits and vegetables, including leafy greens and wheatgrass
- Quieter than centrifugal juicers

Cons:

- Slower than centrifugal juicers
- More expensive than centrifugal juicers
- Can be more difficult to clean

Commercial Juicers:

Commercial juicers are designed for use in commercial settings, such as restaurants, cafes, and juice bars. These juicers are typically larger and more durable than home juicers, and they can handle a higher volume of produce. Commercial juicers come in a variety of types, including centrifugal, masticating, and hydraulic press juicers.

Pros:

- Can handle a higher volume of produce
- Durable and designed for commercial use
- Available in a variety of types

Cons:

- More expensive than home juicers
- Large and require a lot of space
- Not practical for home use

Manual Juicers:

Manual juicers are designed to be operated by hand, without the use of electricity. These juicers come in a variety of types, including citrus juicers and hand-cranked juicers. They are typically less expensive than electric juicers and can be a good option for those who only need to juice small amounts of produce.

Pros:

- Less expensive than electric juicers

- Do not require electricity

- Portable and easy to store

Cons:

- Can be time-consuming to use

- Limited capacity

- Limited versatility

Pulp Ejection Juicers:

Pulp ejection juicers are similar to centrifugal juicers in that they use high-speed spinning to extract juice from produce. However, they also have a mechanism for ejecting the pulp, which allows for continuous juicing without the need to stop and clean out the pulp. Pulp ejection juicers are a good option for those who want to juice large amounts of produce quickly.

Pros:

- Fast and efficient

- Continuous juicing without the need to stop and clean out the pulp

- Can juice most fruits and vegetables

Cons:

- Not as efficient as other juicers

- Can produce a less nutritious juice

- Loud and can create a lot of foam

Combination Juicers:

Combination juicers are designed to be multifunctional, allowing users to juice a variety of produce as well as perform other functions like blending and chopping. These juicers can be more expensive than single-function juicers, but they offer more versatility and can save space in the kitchen.

Pros:

- Versatile and multifunctional

- Save space in the kitchen

- Can perform multiple functions in addition to juicing

Cons:

- More expensive than single-function juicers
- May not be as efficient at juicing as single-function juicers
- More difficult to clean and maintain.

Choosing the Right Ingredients

Juicing is a popular way to consume fruits and vegetables because it allows you to get all the nutrients and vitamins in a concentrated form. However, the quality of the juice depends on the quality of the ingredients used. Using the right ingredients can enhance the flavor and nutritional value of the juice. On the other hand, using poor quality or inappropriate ingredients can lead to a bad taste or poor texture. Additionally, some ingredients may have negative effects on your health if consumed in excess.

Tips for Choosing the Right Ingredients for Juicing:

Choose Fresh and Organic Ingredients:

The quality of the ingredients used in juicing is crucial. It is important to choose fresh, ripe, and organic ingredients whenever possible. Fresh fruits and vegetables contain more nutrients and enzymes than those that have been stored for a long time. Organic produce is free from pesticides and chemicals that can be harmful to your health. When selecting produce, look for those that are firm and free of bruises, mold, or other signs of damage.

Choose a Variety of Colors:

To get the most out of your juice, it is essential to include a variety of colors in your ingredients. Different colors represent different nutrients, so choosing a range of colors ensures that you are getting a wide range of nutrients. For example, red fruits and vegetables contain lycopene, an antioxidant that can protect against cancer and heart disease. Orange and yellow fruits and vegetables are rich in beta-carotene, which is converted into vitamin A in the body. Green leafy vegetables contain chlorophyll, which can help detoxify the body.

Use Seasonal Ingredients:

Using seasonal ingredients in your juice not only ensures freshness but also helps support local agriculture. Seasonal produce is at its peak in terms of flavor and nutrition. It is also cheaper and easier to find when in season. To find out what produce is in season in your area, check with your local farmer's market or produce stand.

Consider the Sugar Content:

While fruits and vegetables are generally considered healthy, some have a higher sugar content than others. It is important to be mindful of the sugar content when choosing ingredients for your juice. High-sugar fruits such as bananas, grapes, and pineapples can cause a rapid increase in blood sugar levels, which can be harmful to people with diabetes or other health conditions. Lower-sugar options such as berries, citrus fruits, and leafy greens are a better choice.

Experiment with Different Combinations:

One of the great things about juicing is that there are endless possibilities when it comes to ingredient combinations. Don't be afraid to experiment with different fruits, vegetables, and herbs to find the perfect combination for your taste buds. Some of the most popular ingredient combinations include:

Green juice: kale, spinach, cucumber, celery, and green apple

Orange juice: carrots, oranges, ginger, and turmeric

Red juice: beets, apples, and carrots

Tropical juice: pineapple, mango, and coconut water

Berry juice: blueberries, strawberries, raspberries, and blackberries

Use the Right Equipment:

To get the most out of your ingredients, it is important to use the right equipment. A high-quality juicer or blender can help extract the maximum amount of nutrients and minimize waste. A centrifugal juicer is a great option for those who want a quick and easy juicing experience, while a masticating juicer is better for those who want to extract the maximum amount of juice from their ingredients. A blender can also be used to make juices, but it may produce a thicker texture than a juicer.

Incorporate Superfoods:

Superfoods are nutrient-dense foods that are considered to be particularly beneficial for health. Adding superfoods to your juice can help boost its nutritional value. Some popular superfoods to consider incorporating into your juice include:

<u>Chia seeds:</u> high in fiber, protein, and omega-3 fatty acids

<u>**Flax seeds:**</u> high in fiber, protein, and omega-3 fatty acids

<u>**Hemp seeds:**</u> high in protein, omega-3 fatty acids, and minerals

<u>**Spirulina:**</u> high in protein, vitamins, and minerals

<u>**Wheatgrass:**</u> high in chlorophyll, vitamins, and minerals

Consider Your Goals:

When choosing ingredients for your juice, it is important to consider your goals. Are you looking to boost your immune system? Improve your digestion? Detoxify your body? Different ingredients have different health benefits, so choosing ingredients that align with your goals can help you achieve better results. For example, if you want to boost your immune system, consider using ingredients such as ginger, turmeric, and citrus fruits.

Preparing Your Produce

Juicing has become an increasingly popular way to consume fruits and vegetables. The health benefits of juicing are well known, as it allows the body to absorb essential nutrients quickly and easily. However, to ensure that you are getting the most out of your juicing experience, it is important to properly prepare your produce before juicing. In this section, we will cover everything you need to know about preparing your produce for juicing, from selecting the right fruits and vegetables to cleaning and storing them.

Selecting Your Produce

The first step in preparing your produce for juicing is selecting the right fruits and vegetables. When choosing produce for juicing, it is important to choose fresh, ripe fruits and vegetables that are high in nutrients. Here are some tips for selecting the best produce for juicing:

1. Choose organic produce when possible. Organic produce is grown without the use of pesticides, which can be harmful to your health.

2. Look for fruits and vegetables that are in season. Seasonal produce is often fresher and more flavorful than produce that is out of season.

3. Choose a variety of fruits and vegetables. To get the most nutritional benefit from your juice, it is important to include a variety of fruits and vegetables in your juice.

4. Choose ripe produce. Ripe produce is easier to juice and will yield more juice than unripe produce.

Cleaning Your Produce

Once you have selected your produce, the next step is to clean it thoroughly. Cleaning your produce is important to remove any dirt, bacteria, or pesticides that may be on the surface of the produce. Here are some tips for cleaning your produce:

1. Rinse your produce under running water. Use cold water to rinse your produce, as hot water can damage the produce.

2. Use a produce brush to clean produce with a thick skin, such as cucumbers or carrots. Scrub the produce with the brush to remove any dirt or debris.

3. Dry your produce with a clean towel or paper towel. Moisture can cause your produce to spoil more quickly, so it is important to dry it thoroughly.

Cutting Your Produce

Once your produce is clean, it is time to cut it into pieces that are small enough to fit into your juicer. The size and shape of the pieces will depend on the type of juicer you have. Here are some tips for cutting your produce:

1. Cut your produce into small pieces. The smaller the pieces, the easier they will be to juice.

2. Cut your produce into pieces that will fit into your juicer. Different juicers have different feed chute sizes, so be sure to check the size of your juicer's feed chute before cutting your produce.

3. Remove any seeds or pits. Some fruits and vegetables, such as apples or cherries, have seeds or pits that need to be removed before juicing.

4. Remove any tough stems or leaves. For example, if juicing kale, you should remove the tough stems and use only the leaves.

Storing Your Produce

Storing your produce properly is important to ensure that it stays fresh and retains its nutritional value. Here are some tips for storing your produce:

1. Store your produce in the refrigerator. Most fruits and vegetables should be stored in the refrigerator to keep them fresh.

2. Store your produce in an airtight container. This will help to keep your produce fresh and prevent it from absorbing any odors from other foods in your refrigerator.

3. Store your produce separately. Some fruits and vegetables produce ethylene gas, which can cause other produce to spoil more quickly. For example, apples should be stored separately from other fruits and vegetables.

4. Use your produce within a few days. Fresh produce can spoil quickly, so it is important to use it within a few days of storing it. If you don't plan

on using your produce right away, consider freezing it to extend its shelf life.

Freezing Your Produce

If you have a surplus of produce that you can't use right away, freezing is a great option to preserve its nutritional value. Freezing can also be a convenient way to have fresh produce on hand for juicing. Here are some tips for freezing your produce:

1. Wash and cut your produce into small pieces.
2. Blanch your produce in boiling water for a few seconds to preserve its color and texture.
3. Place your blanched produce in an airtight container or freezer bag.
4. Label your containers with the date and contents.
5. Freeze your produce for up to six months.
6. Thaw your frozen produce before juicing, and be aware that it may have a slightly different texture than fresh produce.

Tips for Juicing

Juicing is a fantastic way to boost your nutrient intake and achieve a healthier lifestyle. Whether you're new to juicing or an experienced juicer, there are always tips and tricks to learn that can make your juicing experience more enjoyable and effective. Here are some tips for juicing your produce:

Choose the Right Juicer

The first and most important tip for juicing is to choose the right juicer. There are several types of juicers available, including centrifugal, masticating, and citrus juicers. Each type has its own unique features and benefits, so it's important to choose the one that suits your needs and preferences.

Centrifugal juicers are the most common type of juicer and are great for juicing hard fruits and vegetables like

adding different herbs, spices, or sweeteners to your juices to enhance their flavor and nutritional content.

For example, you could add a small amount of honey or maple syrup to your juice for sweetness, or fresh mint or ginger for a refreshing kick. Herbs like basil or parsley can also add a unique flavor and nutrient boost to your juices.

Start Small

If you're new to juicing, it's a good idea to start small and gradually work your way up to larger servings. Drinking too much juice at once can cause digestive issues, so it's important to listen to your body and start with a small serving size.

Aim to start with 4-6 ounces of juice and gradually increase your serving size as your body adjusts. It's also a good idea to drink your juice with a meal or snack to balance out your nutrient intake and prevent blood sugar spikes.

Don't Waste the Pulp

When juicing, the pulp or fiber that's left over can be a valuable source of nutrients and fiber. Don't throw it away! Instead, consider using it in recipes like smoothies, soups, or even baked goods.

You can also add the pulp to your compost pile to enrich your soil and reduce food waste. Just be sure to remove any seeds or tough fibers before using the pulp in your recipes.

Listen to Your Body

Finally, it's important to listen to your body and adjust your juicing routine as needed. Everyone's body is different, and what works for one person may not work for another.

Pay attention to how your body feels after drinking juice and make adjustments as needed. For example, if you experience bloating or digestive discomfort, you may

need to adjust your serving size or the types of produce
you're juicing.

Chapter 4: Recipes for Juices That Boost Immunity

In recent times, there has been a significant increase in the number of individuals seeking ways to boost their immune system. The immune system is responsible for protecting the body against infections and diseases, and a compromised immune system can lead to numerous health complications. One effective way to boost immunity is through consuming healthy and nutritious foods, including juices. Juices made from fresh fruits and vegetables contain essential vitamins and minerals that are vital in supporting the immune system. In this chapter, we will explore some recipes for juices that can help to boost immunity.

Orange, Carrot, and Ginger Juice

There's nothing quite like a refreshing glass of juice to start your day or perk you up in the afternoon. And if you're looking for a juice that's both delicious and healthy, you can't go wrong with orange, carrot, and ginger juice. This vibrant drink is packed with nutrients and vitamins that are essential for optimal health, and it tastes great too! In this section, we'll take a closer look at the benefits of orange, carrot, and ginger juice and provide you with some tips and recipes to help you get the most out of this nutritious beverage.

Why Orange, Carrot, and Ginger Juice?

Orange, carrot, and ginger juice is a popular drink that's packed with essential nutrients that are good for your health. Let's take a closer look at the benefits of each of these ingredients.

Oranges: Oranges are an excellent source of vitamin C, which is essential for a healthy immune system. Vitamin C is also important for the production of collagen, which is necessary for healthy skin and connective tissue. Oranges are also rich in antioxidants, which help to protect your cells from damage caused by free radicals.

Carrots: Carrots are high in beta-carotene, which is converted into vitamin A in the body. Vitamin A is important for maintaining healthy eyesight, skin, and immune function. Carrots are also a good source of fiber, which is important for digestive health.

Ginger: Ginger is a powerful anti-inflammatory agent that can help to reduce inflammation throughout the body. It's also a natural pain reliever and can be helpful for people suffering from arthritis or other inflammatory conditions. Ginger is also a natural digestive aid and can help to relieve nausea and indigestion.

When combined, these three ingredients make a potent and delicious juice that's packed with essential nutrients and health benefits.

Benefits of Orange, Carrot, and Ginger Juice

Here are some of the top benefits of drinking orange, carrot, and ginger juice:

1. **Boosts Immune Function:** The vitamin C in oranges and the beta-carotene in carrots are both important for a healthy immune system. Drinking orange, carrot, and ginger juice can help to boost your immune function and protect your body against illness and disease.

2. **Promotes Healthy Skin:** Vitamin C is essential for the production of collagen, which is necessary for healthy skin. Drinking orange, carrot, and ginger juice can help to improve the appearance of your skin and promote healthy aging.

3. **Reduces Inflammation:** Ginger is a powerful anti-inflammatory agent that can help to reduce inflammation throughout the body. Drinking orange, carrot, and ginger juice can be helpful for people suffering from arthritis or other inflammatory conditions.

4. **Improves Digestion:** Ginger is a natural digestive aid that can help to relieve nausea, indigestion, and other digestive issues. Drinking orange, carrot, and ginger juice can help to promote healthy digestion and reduce digestive discomfort.

5. **Supports Eye Health:** Beta-carotene is converted into vitamin A in the body, which is important for maintaining healthy eyesight. Drinking orange, carrot, and ginger juice can help to promote healthy vision and protect against age-related eye diseases.

6. **Detoxifies the Body:** Oranges, carrots, and ginger all contain compounds that can help to detoxify

the body and promote healthy liver function. Drinking orange, carrot, and ginger juice can help to flush toxins from your body and improve your overall health.

Recipes for Orange, Carrot, and Ginger Juice

Ingredients:

- 4 large carrots, peeled and chopped
- 3 oranges, peeled and segmented
- 1 inch piece of fresh ginger, peeled and chopped

Instructions:

1. Wash and prepare the ingredients.
2. Add the carrots, oranges, and ginger to a juicer and process until smooth.
3. Pour the juice into a glass and serve immediately.

Pineapple, Cucumber, and Mint Juice

The combination of pineapple, cucumber, and mint juice may sound unconventional, but this refreshing beverage is packed with nutrients and offers a range of health benefits. Pineapple is known for its anti-inflammatory properties and ability to aid digestion, while cucumber is rich in hydration and can help flush out toxins from the body. Mint, on the other hand, provides a refreshing flavor and has been used for centuries to help soothe upset stomachs and improve digestion. Let's take a closer look at the nutritional value and health benefits of pineapple, cucumber, and mint juice, before providing you with some delicious and easy-to-make recipes for you to try at home.

Nutritional Value of Pineapple, Cucumber, and Mint

Pineapple:

Pineapple is a tropical fruit that's packed with vitamins, minerals, and enzymes that can help boost your overall health. Here are some of the key nutrients found in pineapple:

1. **Vitamin C:** Pineapple is an excellent source of vitamin C, which is a powerful antioxidant that can help protect your body against free radicals and boost your immune system.
2. **Bromelain:** Pineapple contains a unique enzyme called bromelain, which has anti-inflammatory properties and can help improve digestion.
3. **Fiber:** Pineapple is a good source of dietary fiber, which can help regulate your digestion and keep you feeling full for longer.
4. **Manganese:** Pineapple is also a good source of manganese, which is important for bone health,

wound healing, and the metabolism of carbohydrates and fats.

Cucumber:

Cucumber is a low-calorie, high-water content vegetable that's packed with nutrients. Here are some of the key nutrients found in cucumber:

1. **Hydration:** Cucumber is made up of 96% water, making it an excellent hydrating food that can help keep you cool and refreshed on hot days.

2. **Vitamin K:** Cucumber is a good source of vitamin K, which is important for bone health and blood clotting.

3. **Potassium:** Cucumber is also a good source of potassium, which is important for regulating blood pressure and maintaining fluid balance in the body.

4. **Antioxidants:** Cucumber contains antioxidants like beta-carotene and flavonoids, which can help

protect your body against free radicals and inflammation.

Mint:

Mint is a herb that's been used for centuries for its refreshing flavor and medicinal properties. Here are some of the key nutrients found in mint:

1. **Menthol:** Mint contains a compound called menthol, which has a cooling and soothing effect on the body and can help alleviate nausea and indigestion.
2. **Antioxidants:** Mint contains antioxidants like rosmarinic acid and flavonoids, which can help protect your body against oxidative stress and inflammation.
3. **Vitamin C:** Mint is a good source of vitamin C, which is important for immune function and collagen production.

4. **Fiber:** Mint also contains small amounts of dietary fiber, which can help regulate digestion and promote feelings of fullness.

Health Benefits of Pineapple, Cucumber, and Mint Juice

Aids digestion:

The combination of pineapple, cucumber, and mint in a juice form can help improve digestion and relieve digestive issues like bloating, constipation, and indigestion. Pineapple contains bromelain, which is a natural digestive enzyme that can help break down proteins and improve nutrient absorption. Cucumber is high in water and fiber, which can help promote regular bowel movements and prevent constipation. Mint can help soothe the stomach and alleviate nausea, making it a great ingredient for those with a sensitive digestive system.

Boosts Immunity:

Pineapple, cucumber, and mint are all rich in vitamins and minerals that can help boost your immune system and keep you healthy.

Pineapple is an excellent source of Vitamin C, which is a powerful antioxidant that boosts the immune system. Cucumber and Mint also contain Vitamin C, which helps to promote a healthy immune system. Drinking Pineapple, Cucumber, and Mint Juice can help boost the immune system and prevent illnesses.

Reduces Inflammation:

Pineapple contains bromelain, which has anti-inflammatory properties that can help reduce inflammation in the body. Cucumber and Mint also have anti-inflammatory properties that can help alleviate inflammation. Drinking Pineapple, Cucumber, and Mint Juice can help reduce inflammation in the body and prevent chronic diseases.

Promotes Weight Loss:

Cucumber is a low-calorie vegetable that contains fiber, which helps to keep you full for longer. Mint has a calming effect on the body, which can help reduce stress eating. Drinking Pineapple, Cucumber, and Mint Juice can help promote weight loss by reducing appetite and promoting healthy eating habits.

Promotes Hydration:

Pineapple, Cucumber, and Mint are all excellent sources of water, which makes this juice an excellent source of hydration. Drinking this juice can help keep the body hydrated and prevent dehydration.

Recipes for Pineapple, Cucumber, and Mint Juice

Recipe 1: Pineapple, Cucumber, and Mint Juice

Ingredients:

- 1 cup pineapple, chopped
- 1 cucumber, chopped

- 1/4 cup fresh mint leaves

- 1 cup water

- 1 tablespoon honey (optional)

Directions:

1. Add the chopped pineapple, cucumber, and mint leaves to a blender.

2. Pour in the water and blend until the mixture is smooth.

3. If you'd like your juice sweeter, add honey to taste and blend again.

4. Pour the juice into a glass, add ice if desired, and serve.

Recipe 2: Pineapple, Cucumber, and Mint Juice with Lime

Ingredients:

- 1/2 medium pineapple, peeled and chopped

- 1 medium cucumber, chopped

- 1/4 cup fresh mint leaves

- 1 lime, juiced

- 1 cup water

- 1 tablespoon agave nectar (optional)

Directions:

1. Add the chopped pineapple, cucumber, mint leaves, and lime juice to a blender.

2. Pour in the water and blend until the mixture is smooth.

3. If you'd like your juice sweeter, add agave nectar to taste and blend again.

4. Pour the juice into a glass, add ice if desired, and serve.

Recipe 3: Pineapple, Cucumber, and Mint Juice with Ginger

Ingredients:

- 1/2 medium pineapple, peeled and chopped

- 1 medium cucumber, chopped

- 1/4 cup fresh mint leaves

- 1 tablespoon fresh ginger, grated

- 1 cup water

- 1 tablespoon maple syrup (optional)

Directions:

1. Add the chopped pineapple, cucumber, mint leaves, and grated ginger to a blender.

2. Pour in the water and blend until the mixture is smooth.

3. If you'd like your juice sweeter, add maple syrup to taste and blend again.

4. Pour the juice into a glass, add ice if desired, and serve.

Turmeric and Lemon Juice

Turmeric and lemon juice are two powerful ingredients that have been used for centuries in various traditional medicine practices. Both ingredients have been known to provide numerous health benefits and are often used together in recipes for their combined effects. We will explore the benefits of turmeric and lemon juice, as well as provide some amazing recipes that you can try out.

Benefits of Turmeric

Turmeric is a spice that has been used for thousands of years in traditional medicine practices. It is known for its vibrant yellow color and distinct flavor. Turmeric contains an active ingredient called curcumin, which has been shown to have numerous health benefits.

1. **Anti-inflammatory properties:** Curcumin has been shown to have strong anti-inflammatory properties, which can help reduce inflammation in

the body. Chronic inflammation has been linked to numerous health problems such as heart disease, cancer, and diabetes.

2. **Antioxidant properties:** Turmeric is also a powerful antioxidant, which means it can help protect the body from free radical damage. Free radicals are unstable molecules that can damage cells and contribute to the development of diseases such as cancer.

3. **Improved brain function:** Curcumin has been shown to improve brain function and reduce the risk of cognitive decline. It has also been shown to improve memory and concentration.

4. **Reduced risk of heart disease:** Curcumin has been shown to improve heart health by reducing inflammation and improving cholesterol levels.

5. **Pain relief:** Turmeric has been used for centuries as a natural pain reliever. Curcumin has been

shown to have similar effects to over-the-counter pain relievers such as ibuprofen.

Benefits of Lemon Juice

Lemon juice is a popular ingredient in many recipes and has been used for centuries for its health benefits. Lemon juice is rich in vitamin C, which is an essential nutrient for the body. It also contains other beneficial compounds such as flavonoids and citric acid.

1. **Boosts immune system:** Lemon juice is a great source of vitamin C, which is important for the immune system. Vitamin C helps protect the body from infections and illnesses.

2. **Aids digestion:** Lemon juice has been shown to improve digestion and reduce bloating. It can also help relieve constipation.

3. **Alkalizes the body:** Although lemon juice is acidic, it has an alkalizing effect on the body. This means

that it can help balance the pH levels in the body and reduce the risk of diseases such as cancer.

4. **Promotes hydration:** Lemon juice is a great source of hydration and can help prevent dehydration. It is also a great alternative to sugary drinks.

5. **Promotes healthy skin:** The vitamin C and other compounds in lemon juice can help promote healthy skin. Lemon juice can also help reduce acne and improve the appearance of scars.

Turmeric and Lemon Juice Recipe

Ingredients:

- 1 cup of water
- 1 teaspoon of turmeric powder
- Juice from half a lemon

Instructions:

1. Boil water in a pot.

2. Add turmeric powder to the boiling water and stir.

3. Let the water cool for a few minutes.

4. Add lemon juice to the water and stir.

5. Enjoy!

Beet, Apple, and Carrot Juice

Juicing has become a popular way of consuming fruits and vegetables, providing an easy and delicious way to consume essential nutrients. Three of the most popular ingredients used in juicing are beets, apples, and carrots. These three ingredients are not only delicious but also provide a range of health benefits, including boosting immunity, reducing inflammation, and improving heart health.

Health benefits of Beet, Apple, and Carrot Juice

Beet, apple, and carrot juice are not only delicious but also provide a range of health benefits. Here are some of the key health benefits of each of these ingredients:

Beets:

Beets are packed with essential vitamins and minerals, including vitamin C, vitamin B6, folate, and potassium. They are also rich in antioxidants and phytonutrients, such as betalains, which help fight inflammation and improve heart health. Some of the key health benefits of beets include:

1. **Lowering blood pressure:** Beets are rich in nitrates, which help dilate blood vessels and improve blood flow. This can help lower blood pressure and reduce the risk of heart disease.

2. **Improving exercise performance:** Beets can also improve exercise performance by increasing endurance and reducing fatigue.

3. Boosting brain function: The nitrates in beets also improve blood flow to the brain, which can boost cognitive function and reduce the risk of cognitive decline.

Apples:

Apples are a great source of fiber, vitamin C, and antioxidants. They are also low in calories and can help regulate blood sugar levels. Some of the key health benefits of apples include:

1. **Reducing the risk of heart disease:** Apples are rich in flavonoids, which have been shown to reduce the risk of heart disease by lowering cholesterol levels and improving blood flow.

2. **Boosting immunity:** Apples are also rich in vitamin C, which helps boost immunity and fight infections.

3. **Improving gut health:** Apples are a great source of fiber, which can improve digestive health and reduce the risk of colon cancer.

Carrots:

Carrots are a great source of vitamin A, which is essential for vision health. They are also rich in antioxidants and can help reduce inflammation. Some of the key health benefits of carrots include:

1. **Improving vision health:** Carrots are rich in beta-carotene, which the body converts into vitamin A. Vitamin A is essential for vision health and can help reduce the risk of age-related macular degeneration.

2. **Boosting immunity:** Carrots are also rich in vitamin C, which helps boost immunity and fight infections.

3. **Reducing the risk of cancer:** Carrots contain compounds called polyacetylenes, which have been shown to reduce the risk of cancer by inhibiting the growth of cancer cells.

Recipe:

Ingredients:

- 1 medium-sized beet, peeled and chopped
- 2 medium-sized carrots, peeled and chopped
- 1 medium-sized apple, chopped
- 1-inch piece of ginger, peeled and chopped

- 1 lemon, juiced

Instructions:

1. Wash and prepare all the ingredients.
2. Run the beet, carrots, apple, and ginger through a juicer.
3. Add the lemon juice and stir well.
4. Serve immediately.

Chapter 5: Recipes for Juices That Promote Wellness

Juicing has become increasingly popular in recent years due to the numerous health benefits it provides. Juicing can help improve digestion, boost the immune system, and promote overall wellness. By incorporating fresh fruits and vegetables into your diet, you can reap the benefits of their vitamins, minerals, and other nutrients in an easy-to-digest format. In this chapter, we will be sharing some recipes for juices that promote wellness, which you can easily make at home with a juicer or blender.

Green Goddess Juice

Green Goddess juice is a popular green juice that has gained a lot of popularity in recent years. The juice is made from a variety of green vegetables and fruits, and it is rich in nutrients that provide numerous health benefits. It is a refreshing and delicious way to get your daily dose of vitamins and minerals.

Benefits of Green Goddess Juice:

Green Goddess juice is packed with vitamins, minerals, and antioxidants, making it an excellent choice for maintaining good health. Here are some of the benefits of Green Goddess juice:

Boosts Immunity:

Green Goddess juice is loaded with nutrients that are essential for maintaining a healthy immune system. The juice is rich in vitamin C, which is known for its immune-boosting properties. It also contains vitamin A, which is essential for maintaining healthy skin, mucous membranes, and the immune system.

Detoxifies the Body:

Green Goddess juice is a great way to detoxify your body. The juice is loaded with chlorophyll, which helps to cleanse the liver and remove toxins from the body. It also contains antioxidants, which help to protect the body from free radicals that can cause damage to the cells.

Promotes Weight Loss:

Green Goddess juice is a great way to lose weight. The juice is low in calories and high in fiber, which helps to keep you feeling full and satisfied for longer periods. It also contains ingredients that help to boost metabolism, which can help to burn fat and promote weight loss.

Improves Digestion:

Green Goddess juice is an excellent source of fiber, which helps to improve digestion. The juice also contains digestive enzymes that help to break down food and absorb nutrients more efficiently.

Boosts Energy:

Green Goddess juice is a great way to boost your energy levels. The juice is loaded with vitamins and minerals that help to support energy production in the body. It also contains natural sugars that provide a quick burst of energy.

Green Goddess juice recipe

Ingredients:

- 1 green apple
- 1/2 cucumber
- 1/2 lemon, peeled
- 2 handfuls of spinach

- 1 inch piece of ginger root

- 1/2 cup of fresh mint leaves

- 1/2 cup of fresh parsley leaves

- 1/2 cup of coconut water

Instructions:

1. Wash all the fruits and vegetables thoroughly.

2. Cut the green apple and cucumber into small pieces, and remove the seeds.

3. Peel the ginger and lemon, and cut them into small pieces.

4. Add all the ingredients into a blender, and blend until smooth.

5. If the mixture is too thick, add a little more coconut water to thin it out to your desired consistency.

6. Pour the Green Goddess juice into a glass, and enjoy!

Blueberry and Kale Juice

Blueberry and kale juice is an amazing combination of two superfoods that provides a plethora of health benefits. Kale is a cruciferous vegetable that is rich in vitamins A, C, K, and minerals such as calcium, magnesium, and iron. Blueberries are loaded with antioxidants, fiber, and vitamin C. Together, these two ingredients make a delicious and nutritious juice that can help boost your immune system, support healthy digestion, and promote overall wellness.

The Benefits of Blueberry and Kale Juice

Boosts Immune System

Blueberry and kale juice are both rich in antioxidants, which help fight free radicals that damage cells and weaken the immune system. The vitamin C in blueberries and kale also helps support the immune system by increasing the production of white blood cells.

Supports Healthy Digestion

Kale is an excellent source of fiber, which promotes healthy digestion and regular bowel movements. Blueberries also contain fiber, which helps keep the digestive system running smoothly. Drinking blueberry and kale juice can help keep your gut healthy and reduce the risk of digestive problems.

Promotes Heart Health

Blueberry and kale juice are both good for the heart. Kale contains compounds that help lower cholesterol levels and reduce the risk of heart disease. Blueberries are rich in flavonoids, which help improve blood flow and reduce inflammation in the arteries.

May Help Reduce Cancer Risk

Kale and blueberries both contain compounds that have been shown to have anti-cancer properties. The antioxidants in blueberries and the phytochemicals in kale can help prevent cancer cells from forming and spreading.

Improves Brain Function

Blueberries are known as a brain food because of their high levels of antioxidants. Kale also contains compounds that have been shown to improve cognitive function. Drinking blueberry and kale juice can help boost brain function and improve memory.

Recipe:

Ingredients:

- 2 cups of kale
- 1 cup of blueberries
- 1 apple
- 1 lemon

Instructions:

1. Wash the kale, blueberries, apple, and lemon.

2. Cut the apple into small pieces and remove the core.

3. Cut the lemon into quarters.

4. Add the kale, blueberries, apple, and lemon to a juicer.

5. Juice the ingredients until smooth.

6. Pour the juice into a glass and enjoy!

Watermelon and Lime Juice

Watermelon and lime juice is a refreshing and delicious combination that is perfect for a hot summer day. This bright and flavorful drink is packed with vitamins, minerals, and antioxidants that can provide a host of health benefits.

Together, watermelon and lime create a powerhouse of nutrients that can provide a range of health benefits. In addition to their nutritional value, both fruits are also high in water content, which can help keep you hydrated and support healthy digestion.

Benefits of Watermelon and Lime Juice

Before we dive into the recipes, let's take a look at some of the benefits of watermelon and lime juice. Watermelon is a hydrating fruit that is rich in vitamins A and C, as well as antioxidants. It is also low in calories and has a high water content, making it an excellent choice for those looking to lose weight or maintain a healthy diet. Lime, on the other hand, is rich in vitamin C and has anti-inflammatory properties that can help reduce the risk of chronic diseases such as cancer and heart disease. The combination of these two fruits creates a healthy and delicious drink that is perfect for anyone looking to improve their overall health.

Recipe:

Ingredients:

- 4 cups of watermelon chunks
- 2 limes, juiced
- 2 cups of cold water
- 2 tbsp of honey (optional)
- Ice cubes

Instructions:

1. Add the watermelon chunks and lime juice to a blender and blend until smooth.

2. Strain the mixture through a fine-mesh strainer into a pitcher.

3. Add the cold water and honey (if using) to the pitcher and stir until combined.

4. Serve the juice over ice and enjoy!

Pomegranate and Cranberry Juice

Pomegranate and cranberry juice is a delicious and refreshing drink that is packed with health benefits. This juice recipe is perfect for those who want to add more antioxidants, vitamins, and minerals to their diet.

Pomegranate and cranberry juice are two of the most popular superfoods that are known for their health benefits. These two fruits are rich in antioxidants, which help protect the body from harmful free radicals. They are also high in vitamins and minerals, such as vitamin C, vitamin K, and potassium, which support overall health and wellbeing.

Benefits of Pomegranate and Cranberry Juice

1. **Rich in Antioxidants:** Both pomegranate and cranberry are loaded with antioxidants, which help to protect the body from oxidative stress. Oxidative stress occurs when there is an

imbalance between free radicals and antioxidants in the body. This imbalance can lead to cell damage and contribute to the development of chronic diseases such as cancer, heart disease, and Alzheimer's disease.

2. **Anti-inflammatory Properties:** Pomegranate and cranberry juice are also known for their anti-inflammatory properties. Chronic inflammation is linked to the development of many diseases, including arthritis, diabetes, and heart disease. The antioxidants in pomegranate and cranberry juice can help to reduce inflammation in the body, which may help to prevent these conditions.

3. **Boosts Heart Health:** Studies have shown that both pomegranate and cranberry juice can help to lower blood pressure and cholesterol levels, which are risk factors for heart disease. The antioxidants in these fruits may also help to reduce the buildup

of plaque in the arteries, which can lead to a heart attack or stroke.

4. **May Help Prevent Cancer:** Some studies have suggested that the antioxidants in pomegranate and cranberry juice may have cancer-fighting properties. In particular, they may help to prevent the growth and spread of breast, prostate, and colon cancer cells.

5. **May Improve Brain Function:** Preliminary research has suggested that drinking pomegranate and cranberry juice may improve brain function in older adults. This is thought to be due to the high levels of antioxidants in these fruits, which may help to protect the brain from oxidative stress and inflammation.

Now, let's move on to the recipe.

Pomegranate and Cranberry Juice Recipe

Ingredients:

- 1 cup fresh cranberries
- 1 cup pomegranate seeds
- 1/4 cup honey
- 4 cups water

Instructions:

1. Rinse the cranberries and remove any stems.
2. Cut open the pomegranate and remove the seeds.
3. Add the cranberries, pomegranate seeds, honey, and water to a blender.
4. Blend on high until the mixture is smooth.
5. Strain the mixture through a fine mesh strainer into a pitcher.
6. Chill the juice in the refrigerator for at least one hour.
7. Serve and enjoy!

Tips:

1. You can adjust the sweetness of the juice by adding more or less honey, depending on your preference.

2. To make the juice more tart, you can add a squeeze of fresh lemon or lime juice.

3. If you don't have a blender, you can also use a food processor or a juicer.

4. You can also freeze the juice into ice cubes and use them to chill other drinks, such as sparkling water or cocktails.

Chapter 6: Recipes for Juices That Fight Cancer

Cancer is the second leading cause of death globally, responsible for an estimated 9.6 million deaths in 2018 alone. While there is no known cure for cancer, various studies have shown that a healthy diet can reduce the risk of developing cancer or even help fight the disease. One of the ways to achieve this is by consuming juices that contain cancer-fighting ingredients.

In this chapter, we will explore 4 juice recipes that are not only delicious but also packed with nutrients that can help fight cancer. We will discuss their health benefits, the ingredient used and their recipes.

Carrot, Ginger, and Turmeric Juice

Carrot, ginger, and turmeric juice is a delicious and nutritious beverage that has gained popularity in recent years for its numerous health benefits. This juice is made by combining fresh carrots, ginger root, and turmeric root in a juicer or blender. The resulting juice is a vibrant orange color and has a unique flavor that is both sweet and spicy.

Health Benefits of Carrot, Ginger, and Turmeric Juice:

1. **Anti-inflammatory properties:** Turmeric and ginger both contain powerful anti-inflammatory compounds, which can help reduce inflammation throughout the body. Chronic inflammation is linked to a wide range of health problems, including heart disease, cancer, and Alzheimer's disease.

2. **Immune-boosting properties:** Carrots are rich in vitamin C, which is essential for a healthy immune system. Ginger and turmeric also have immune-boosting properties, which can help prevent colds, flu, and other infections.

3. **Digestive health:** Ginger is well-known for its ability to soothe upset stomachs and relieve nausea. Carrots contain fiber, which can help promote healthy digestion and prevent constipation.

4. **Heart health:** Carrots are rich in potassium, which can help lower blood pressure and reduce the risk of heart disease. Turmeric also has heart-protective properties, which can help reduce the risk of heart attacks and strokes.

5. **Cancer prevention:** Turmeric contains a compound called curcumin, which has been shown to have anti-cancer properties. Carrots also

contain antioxidants, which can help prevent cancer by neutralizing harmful free radicals.

Nutritional Content of Carrot, Ginger, and Turmeric Juice:

Carrots:

Carrots are a rich source of vitamins, minerals, and antioxidants. One cup of chopped carrots (about 128 grams) contains:

- Calories: 52
- Carbohydrates: 12 grams
- Fiber: 4 grams
- Protein: 1 gram
- Fat: 0 grams
- Vitamin A: 428% of the Daily Value (DV)
- Vitamin K: 21% of the DV
- Potassium: 12% of the DV
- Vitamin C: 10% of the DV

Ginger:

Ginger is a root that has been used for medicinal purposes for thousands of years. It is a good source of vitamins, minerals, and antioxidants. One ounce (28 grams) of fresh ginger contains:

- Calories: 20
- Carbohydrates: 5 grams
- Fiber: 1 gram
- Protein: 0 grams
- Fat: 0 grams
- Vitamin B6: 2% of the DV
- Iron: 1% of the DV
- Magnesium: 1% of the DV

Turmeric:

Turmeric is a bright yellow root that is a member of the ginger family. It is a potent anti-inflammatory agent and has been used for thousands of years in traditional medicine. One tablespoon (6 grams) of ground turmeric contains:

- Calories: 24
- Carbohydrates: 4 grams
- Fiber: 2 grams
- Protein: 1 gram
- Fat: 0 grams
- Iron: 16% of the DV
- Potassium: 3% of the DV
- Vitamin C: 3% of the DV

Recipe:

Ingredients:

- 4 large carrots, peeled and chopped
- 1 inch piece of fresh ginger, peeled and chopped
- 1 teaspoon of ground turmeric
- 1 lemon, juiced

Instructions:

1. Add the carrots, ginger, and turmeric to a juicer and juice until smooth.
2. Pour the juice into a glass and add the lemon juice.
3. Stir well and enjoy!

Green Tea and Apple Juice

Green tea and apple juice are two beverages that have become increasingly popular in recent years, and for good reason. Both have numerous health benefits and are refreshing, tasty drinks that can be enjoyed at any time of day.

Health Benefits of Green Tea

Green tea is packed with antioxidants, which are compounds that help to protect the body from damage caused by free radicals. Free radicals are unstable molecules that can damage cells and contribute to the development of chronic diseases, such as cancer and heart disease.

One of the most well-known antioxidants in green tea is epigallocatechin gallate (EGCG), which has been shown to have a wide range of health benefits. These include:

1. **Reducing the risk of cardiovascular disease:** Studies have shown that drinking green tea can help to lower blood pressure and cholesterol levels, which are two major risk factors for heart disease.

2. **Improving brain function:** Green tea contains caffeine, which is a natural stimulant that can help to improve alertness and cognitive function. It also contains an amino acid called L-theanine, which has a calming effect and can help to reduce stress and anxiety.

3. **Preventing certain types of cancer:** EGCG has been shown to have anticancer properties and may help to prevent the development of certain types of cancer, such as breast, lung, and prostate cancer.

4. **Promoting weight loss:** Green tea has been shown to increase metabolism and promote fat

burning, which can help to support weight loss efforts.

Health Benefits of Apple Juice

Like green tea, apple juice is also rich in antioxidants. It is also a good source of vitamins and minerals, including vitamin C, potassium, and folate. Some of the health benefits of apple juice include:

1. **Boosting the immune system:** Apple juice contains vitamin C, which is important for a healthy immune system. It also contains other antioxidants, which can help to protect the body from damage caused by free radicals.

2. **Improving digestion:** Apple juice contains soluble fiber, which can help to promote healthy digestion and prevent constipation.

3. **Lowering the risk of certain diseases:** Studies have shown that consuming apples and apple juice may help to reduce the risk of certain

diseases, such as Alzheimer's disease, asthma, and certain types of cancer.

4. **Promoting hydration:** Apple juice is a good source of water and can help to promote hydration. This is important for maintaining healthy skin, preventing fatigue, and supporting overall health and wellbeing.

Green Tea and Apple Juice recipe:

Ingredients:

- 2 cups of water
- 2 green tea bags
- 1 cup of apple juice
- Honey or sugar (optional)
- Ice cubes (optional)

Instructions:

1. Bring 2 cups of water to a boil in a pot or kettle.

2. Remove the pot or kettle from heat and add 2 green tea bags to the water.

3. Let the tea steep for 2-3 minutes.

4. Remove the tea bags and let the tea cool to room temperature.

5. In a separate container, pour 1 cup of apple juice.

6. If desired, add honey or sugar to the apple juice to sweeten it.

7. Once the tea has cooled, add it to the apple juice and stir.

8. If desired, add ice cubes to the mixture to chill it.

Cabbage and Carrot Juice

Cabbage and carrot juice is a delicious and nutritious drink that offers numerous health benefits. This refreshing beverage is easy to make, and it's a great way to start your day or give yourself a boost of energy throughout the day.

Health Benefits of Cabbage and Carrot Juice

Cabbage and carrot juice is a nutrient-packed drink that can provide numerous health benefits. Here are some of the top benefits of this delicious beverage:

1. **Boosts Immunity:** Cabbage and carrot juice is an excellent source of vitamin C, which is essential for a healthy immune system. This vitamin helps to protect against infections and diseases, and it also helps to promote the production of white blood cells.

Promotes Digestive Health: Both cabbage and carrots are rich in fiber, which is essential for healthy digestion. Drinking cabbage and carrot juice can help to promote regular bowel movements and reduce the risk of constipation.

2. **Reduces Inflammation:** Cabbage contains compounds called anthocyanins, which have anti-inflammatory properties. These compounds help to reduce inflammation in the body and can help to alleviate symptoms of arthritis and other inflammatory conditions.

3. **Supports Heart Health:** Carrots contain high levels of potassium, which can help to lower blood pressure and reduce the risk of heart disease. Cabbage also contains compounds that can help to lower cholesterol levels, further supporting heart health.

Promotes Healthy Skin: Cabbage and carrot juice is rich in antioxidants, which help to protect the skin from damage caused by free radicals. These antioxidants can help to reduce the appearance of fine lines and wrinkles, and can also help to prevent skin damage caused by UV radiation.

Cabbage and Carrot Juice Recipe

Now that you know about the benefits of cabbage and carrot juice, let's get into the recipe. Here's what you'll need:

Ingredients:

- 1/2 head of green cabbage
- 4 large carrots
- 1/2 inch piece of ginger
- 1 lemon

Instructions:

1. Wash the cabbage and carrots thoroughly.
2. Cut the cabbage into quarters and remove the core. Cut the quarters into smaller pieces.

3. Peel the carrots and cut them into smaller pieces.

4. Peel the ginger and cut it into small pieces.

5. Juice the cabbage, carrots, and ginger using a juicer.

6. Squeeze the lemon into the juice and stir well.

7. Pour the juice into a glass and enjoy!

Spinach and Lemon Juice

Spinach and Lemon Juice Recipe is one of the healthiest and most delicious drinks that you can prepare at home. This recipe is full of essential nutrients and vitamins that are beneficial for the overall health of the body. It is a perfect recipe for those who want to stay fit and healthy. This recipe is easy to prepare and requires only a few ingredients, making it an ideal choice for busy individuals who are always on the go.

Benefits of Spinach and Lemon Juice

Spinach and lemon juice are packed with essential vitamins and minerals that are good for the body. Here are some of the benefits of consuming spinach and lemon juice:

1. **Boosts Immunity:** Spinach is loaded with vitamin C, which helps to boost the immune system. The

antioxidants in spinach help to protect the body against diseases and infections.

2. **Improves Digestion:** Lemon juice is rich in citric acid, which helps to stimulate the production of digestive juices. This aids in the digestion of food and prevents bloating and constipation.

3. **Enhances Heart Health:** Spinach is rich in potassium and magnesium, which are essential for maintaining a healthy heart. Lemon juice also helps to regulate blood pressure and reduces the risk of heart diseases.

4. **Promotes Weight Loss:** Spinach is low in calories and high in fiber, making it an ideal food for weight loss. Lemon juice also helps to boost metabolism and aids in burning fat.

5. **Improves Bone Health:** Spinach is rich in calcium, which is essential for strong bones. The vitamin C in lemon juice also helps to absorb calcium in the body.

6. **Aids in Detoxification:** Spinach and lemon juice are natural detoxifiers that help to eliminate toxins from the body. This helps to keep the body healthy and prevents diseases.

Step-by-Step Guide to Making Spinach and Lemon Juice

Now that we know the benefits of spinach and lemon juice, let us take a look at how to make this delicious recipe. Here are the step-by-step instructions:

Ingredients:

- 2 cups of fresh spinach leaves
- 1 lemon
- 1/2 cup of water
- 1 teaspoon of honey
- Ice cubes (optional)

Instructions:

1. Wash the spinach leaves thoroughly and remove any dirt or debris. Place the leaves in a blender.

2. Cut the lemon in half and squeeze the juice into the blender.

3. Add 1/2 cup of water to the blender.

4. Add 1 teaspoon of honey to the blender.

5. Blend all the ingredients together until the mixture is smooth.

6. If you prefer your drink to be cold, add some ice cubes to the blender and blend for a few seconds.

7. Pour the mixture into a glass and enjoy your delicious and healthy spinach and lemon juice.

Tips:

1. You can add more or less honey to the recipe depending on your preference.

2. You can also add other ingredients such as ginger, mint leaves or cucumber to enhance the flavor of the drink.

3. Use fresh spinach leaves for the best flavor and nutrients.

4. Use a high-powered blender to ensure that the mixture is smooth and well-blended.

Chapter 7: Smoothies for Cancer Patients

Cancer patients often face a challenging time when it comes to eating nutritious and balanced meals. The side effects of cancer treatments such as chemotherapy and radiation can cause various digestive problems and weaken the immune system. However, maintaining a healthy diet is crucial for cancer patients to support their immune system, energy levels, and overall well-being.

One of the best ways to provide essential nutrients to cancer patients is through smoothies. Smoothies are a great way to pack in several servings of fruits, vegetables, and other healthy ingredients into one glass. In this chapter, we will explore some delicious recipes to try along with their health benefits

Berry Blast Smoothie

Smoothies are a great way to start your day with a blast of energy and nutrition. They are easy to make, refreshing, and delicious. One of the most popular smoothies is the berry blast smoothie. This smoothie is not only tasty but also packed with essential vitamins and minerals.

Recipe:

Ingredients:

To make a berry blast smoothie, you will need the following ingredients:

- 1 cup of frozen mixed berries (strawberries, blueberries, raspberries, and blackberries)
- 1 banana
- 1 cup of spinach leaves
- 1 cup of unsweetened almond milk

- 1 tablespoon of chia seeds

- 1 tablespoon of honey (optional)

Directions:

Now that you have gathered all the ingredients, it is time to start making your berry blast smoothie. Follow these steps to make a delicious and healthy smoothie:

Step 1: Add the frozen mixed berries to a blender.

Step 2: Peel the banana and add it to the blender.

Step 3: Add the spinach leaves to the blender.

Step 4: Pour in the almond milk.

Step 5: Add the chia seeds to the blender.

Step 6: If you want your smoothie to be sweeter, add a tablespoon of honey.

Step 7: Blend all the ingredients together until smooth.

Step 8: Pour the smoothie into a glass and enjoy!

Health Benefits of Berry Blast Smoothie

The berry blast smoothie is not only delicious but also packed with essential vitamins and minerals. Here are some of the benefits of drinking a berry blast smoothie:

1. **High in Antioxidants:** Berries are rich in antioxidants, which protect the body from free radicals that can cause damage to cells. By drinking a berry blast smoothie, you can increase your antioxidant intake, which can help reduce the risk of chronic diseases.

2. **Rich in Fiber:** The chia seeds in this smoothie are an excellent source of fiber, which can help regulate digestion and promote satiety. Fiber can also help lower cholesterol levels and reduce the risk of heart disease.

3. **Good for Eye Health:** Spinach is rich in lutein and zeaxanthin, which are essential for eye health. These nutrients can help reduce the risk of age-related macular degeneration and cataracts.

4. **Boosts Immunity:** Berries are also rich in vitamin C, which is essential for a healthy immune system. By drinking a berry blast smoothie, you can increase your vitamin C intake, which can help boost your immunity and fight off infections.

5. **Low in Calories:** The berry blast smoothie is low in calories, making it an excellent choice for those who are watching their weight. This smoothie is also vegan, gluten-free, and dairy-free, making it suitable for those with dietary restrictions.

Peanut Butter and Banana Smoothie

Smoothies have become a popular and healthy way to start the day, snack or mealtime. They are quick, easy, and delicious, making them a go-to option for many people. One smoothie that has gained popularity is the Peanut Butter and Banana Smoothie. This smoothie is not only tasty but also provides numerous health benefits.

Health Benefits:

The Peanut Butter and Banana Smoothie is not only delicious but also packed with numerous health benefits. Here are some benefits of this smoothie:

Rich in Fiber:

Bananas are rich in fiber, which is essential for a healthy digestive system. The fiber in bananas helps to regulate bowel movements, prevent constipation, and reduce the risk of colon cancer.

High in Potassium:

Bananas are also rich in potassium, an essential mineral that helps to regulate blood pressure, reduce the risk of stroke, and improve heart health.

Good Source of Protein:

Peanut butter is an excellent source of protein, which is essential for building and repairing tissues in the body. Protein also helps to boost metabolism, reduce hunger, and promote weight loss.

High in Healthy Fats:

Peanut butter is high in healthy fats such as monounsaturated and polyunsaturated fats, which are essential for brain health, reducing inflammation, and improving heart health.

Contains Antioxidants:

Cinnamon, which is a common ingredient in Peanut Butter and Banana Smoothies, is rich in antioxidants, which help to fight inflammation, reduce the risk of chronic diseases, and improve brain function.

Recipe:

Ingredients:

- 1 banana, peeled and chopped
- 2 tablespoons of peanut butter
- 1 cup of unsweetened almond milk
- 1 teaspoon of honey (optional)
- 1 cup of ice cubes

Instructions:

1. Add the chopped banana, peanut butter, almond milk, and honey (if using) to a blender.
2. Blend on high speed until the mixture is smooth and creamy.
3. Add the ice cubes to the blender and blend again until the smoothie is thick and icy.

4. Pour the smoothie into a glass and enjoy
immediately.

Chocolate Avocado Smoothie

Smoothies have become a popular breakfast and snack option for many people around the world. They are easy to make, customizable, and packed with nutrients that can help you feel energized and satisfied throughout the day. One smoothie recipe that has gained a lot of attention in recent years is the Chocolate Avocado Smoothie. This smoothie combines the richness of chocolate with the creaminess of avocado, resulting in a decadent and healthy treat that is perfect for any time of day.

Nutritional Benefits of the Chocolate Avocado Smoothie

The Chocolate Avocado Smoothie is not only delicious but also packed with nutritional benefits that can help you feel your best. Here are just a few of the many benefits of this smoothie:

1. **Healthy Fats:** Avocados are a great source of healthy fats, including monounsaturated and polyunsaturated fats. These fats can help reduce inflammation in the body, improve heart health, and even aid in weight loss.

2. **Antioxidants:** Chocolate is a rich source of antioxidants, which can help protect the body against damage from free radicals. Free radicals are unstable molecules that can damage cells and contribute to the development of chronic diseases.

3. **Fiber:** Avocados are also a good source of fiber, which can help regulate digestion and promote feelings of fullness. This can help prevent overeating and aid in weight loss.

4. **Vitamins and Minerals:** Avocados are packed with vitamins and minerals, including vitamin K, vitamin C, potassium, and magnesium. These

nutrients are important for maintaining overall health and wellness.

5. **Protein:** Many Chocolate Avocado Smoothie recipes also include a source of protein, such as Greek yogurt or protein powder. Protein is important for building and repairing muscle tissue, as well as promoting satiety and preventing overeating.

Recipe:

Ingredients:

- 1 ripe avocado
- 1 banana (frozen or fresh)
- 1 cup almond milk (or any other type of milk)
- 1 tablespoon cocoa powder
- 1-2 tablespoons honey or maple syrup (optional)
- Ice cubes (optional)

Instructions:

1. Cut the avocado in half, remove the pit, and scoop out the flesh into a blender.

2. Add the banana, almond milk, cocoa powder, and sweetener (if using) to the blender.

3. Blend on high speed until smooth and creamy. If the mixture is too thick, add a few ice cubes to thin it out.

4. Taste the smoothie and adjust the sweetness as needed.

5. Pour the smoothie into a glass and enjoy immediately.

Mango and Coconut Milk Smoothie

Smoothies are a perfect way to enjoy a nutritious and delicious meal on-the-go. They are easy to make, require minimal ingredients and can be customized to your taste. Among the plethora of smoothie recipes available, mango and coconut milk smoothie stands out because of its tropical flavors, refreshing taste, and health benefits. Mangoes are loaded with vitamins, minerals, and antioxidants, while coconut milk is rich in healthy fats and nutrients.

Ingredients:

- To make this delicious smoothie, you will need:
- 1 cup of frozen mango chunks
- 1 cup of coconut milk
- 1 ripe banana
- 1 tbsp honey
- 1 tbsp chia seeds (optional)

- 1/4 tsp vanilla extract (optional)

- 1/4 tsp ground cinnamon (optional)

- 1/2 cup ice cubes (optional)

Instructions:

1. Gather all the ingredients and put them into a blender.

2. Blend the ingredients until they are smooth and creamy.

3. Pour the smoothie into a glass and serve immediately.

Benefits:

1. **Promotes Digestive Health:** Mangoes are an excellent source of dietary fiber, which aids digestion and prevents constipation. Coconut milk also contains fiber that promotes digestive health.

2. **Boosts Immune System:** Mangoes are rich in vitamin C and antioxidants, which boost the

immune system and protect the body against infections and diseases.

3. **Supports Heart Health:** Coconut milk contains healthy fats, such as medium-chain triglycerides (MCTs), that improve heart health by lowering cholesterol levels and reducing the risk of heart disease.

4. **Aids in Weight Loss:** Mangoes are low in calories and high in fiber, which makes them an excellent food for weight loss. Coconut milk also contains healthy fats that help in weight management.

5. **Provides Energy:** Mangoes are a rich source of natural sugars, while coconut milk contains medium-chain fatty acids that provide an instant source of energy.

Tips:

1. Use ripe mangoes for a sweeter taste and smoother texture.

2. Use unsweetened coconut milk to reduce sugar content.

3. Add more ice cubes if you prefer a thicker smoothie.

4. Top the smoothie with shredded coconut or sliced mango for a decorative touch.

Chapter 8: Nutritious Snacks for Cancer Patients

Cancer patients often struggle with a loss of appetite, nausea, and fatigue due to the effects of their treatment. This can make it difficult for them to get the nutrients they need to support their immune system, heal, and maintain their strength. However, snacking can be an effective way to get the necessary nutrients into a cancer patient's diet without overwhelming their appetite. Nutritious snacks for cancer patients should be easily digestible, rich in protein and calories, and packed with vitamins and minerals to support their immune system. In this chapter, we will explore some of the best snacks for cancer patients and provide tips on how to make them more appetizing and easy to consume.

Cucumber and Hummus

Cucumber and hummus is a classic combination of fresh, crunchy cucumber and creamy, flavorful hummus that has become a popular appetizer, snack, or light meal in recent years. This dish is not only delicious, but it is also healthy and easy to prepare, making it a go-to choice for anyone looking for a quick and nutritious meal.

Nutritional Benefits of Cucumbers and Hummus

Cucumbers are low in calories and high in water content, making them a great option for those looking to lose weight or maintain a healthy diet. They are also rich in antioxidants, which help protect against oxidative stress and inflammation, and they are a good source of vitamin C and potassium.

Hummus is also a nutritious food, as it is a great source of protein, fiber, and healthy fats. Chickpeas, the main ingredient in hummus, are packed with protein and fiber, which help keep you feeling full and satisfied. Tahini, another key ingredient in hummus, is a rich source of healthy fats, including omega-3 fatty acids, which help support heart health and reduce inflammation.

How to Make Cucumber and Hummus

Making cucumber and hummus is a simple and straightforward process that requires only a few basic ingredients. Here's what you'll need:

- 1 large cucumber
- 1 cup of hummus
- 1 tablespoon of olive oil
- Salt and pepper to taste

Step 1: Prepare the cucumber

Wash the cucumber thoroughly and pat it dry with a clean towel. Cut off the ends of the cucumber and slice it into thin rounds or strips, depending on your preference.

Step 2: Prepare the hummus

If you are making your own hummus, follow your favorite recipe to prepare it. If you are using store-bought hummus, simply open the container and give it a good stir to make sure it is well-mixed.

Step 3: Assemble the dish

Arrange the cucumber slices or strips on a plate or serving dish, leaving some space between them. Spoon the hummus onto the plate, either in the center or around the edges of the cucumber slices. Drizzle the olive oil over the hummus and sprinkle salt and pepper to taste.

Quinoa Salad with Veggies

Quinoa salad with veggies is a delicious, healthy, and easy-to-prepare meal that is perfect for any time of the year. Whether you're looking for a quick lunch, a filling dinner, or a nutritious side dish, this recipe has got you covered. This salad is packed with protein, fiber, vitamins, and minerals, making it a nutritious and satisfying meal option.

Nutritional Benefits:

Quinoa is a highly nutritious food that is rich in protein, fiber, vitamins, and minerals. It is a complete protein, meaning it contains all nine essential amino acids that the body cannot produce on its own. Quinoa is also high in fiber, which can help with digestion, weight management, and reducing the risk of chronic diseases such as heart disease and diabetes. Additionally, quinoa is rich in vitamins and minerals, including iron, magnesium, potassium, and zinc, which are essential for maintaining good health.

The vegetables used in this recipe are also highly nutritious. Bell peppers are rich in vitamin C, which can boost the immune system and support healthy skin. Cucumbers are low in calories and high in water, making them a great option for hydration. Tomatoes are rich in lycopene, an antioxidant that can help protect against cancer and heart disease. Red onions are a good source of fiber and contain compounds that can help lower cholesterol and blood pressure.

Quinoa Salad with Veggies Recipe:

Ingredients:

- 1 cup quinoa
- 2 cups water or vegetable broth
- 1 red bell pepper, chopped
- 1 yellow bell pepper, chopped
- 1 cucumber, chopped

- 2 tomatoes, chopped
- 1/2 red onion, chopped
- 1/4 cup fresh parsley, chopped
- 1/4 cup fresh mint, chopped
- 1/4 cup lemon juice
- 1/4 cup olive oil
- Salt and pepper to taste

Instructions:

1. Rinse the quinoa in a fine-mesh strainer and transfer it to a medium saucepan.
2. Add 2 cups of water or vegetable broth to the saucepan and bring to a boil.
3. Reduce the heat to low, cover the saucepan, and let the quinoa simmer for 15-20 minutes or until all the liquid is absorbed.
4. Remove the quinoa from the heat and let it cool.
5. In a large mixing bowl, combine the chopped bell peppers, cucumber, tomatoes, red onion, parsley, and mint.

6. Add the cooled quinoa to the bowl and mix well.

7. In a small bowl, whisk together the lemon juice, olive oil, salt, and pepper to make the dressing.

8. Pour the dressing over the quinoa salad and toss well to combine.

9. Serve the salad immediately or chill it in the fridge until ready to serve.

Guacamole and Sliced Vegetables

Guacamole and sliced vegetables are a match made in heaven. The creamy, tangy flavor of guacamole pairs perfectly with the fresh, crisp texture of sliced vegetables. Whether you're looking for a healthy snack or a crowd-pleasing appetizer, this recipe is sure to satisfy.

The beauty of guacamole and sliced vegetables is that it's incredibly easy to make. With just a handful of ingredients and a few minutes of prep time, you can have a delicious and nutritious snack.

Ingredients:

- For the guacamole:
- 3 ripe avocados
- 1/4 cup diced red onion
- 1/4 cup diced tomatoes
- 1 jalapeño, seeded and minced

- 2 cloves garlic, minced

- 1/4 cup chopped fresh cilantro

- Juice of 1 lime

- Salt and pepper to taste

- For the sliced vegetables:

- 1 red bell pepper, sliced

- 1 yellow bell pepper, sliced

- 1 cucumber, sliced

- 2 carrots, sliced

- 1 celery stalk, sliced

Instructions:

1. Begin by making the guacamole. Cut the avocados in half and remove the pit. Scoop the flesh into a bowl and mash with a fork.

2. Add the diced red onion, tomatoes, jalapeño, garlic, cilantro, lime juice, salt, and pepper to the bowl. Mix well to combine.

3. Taste the guacamole and adjust the seasoning as necessary.

4. Next, prepare the sliced vegetables. Wash and slice the peppers, cucumber, carrots, and celery into thin strips.

5. Arrange the sliced vegetables on a platter and serve with the guacamole on the side.

6. Enjoy!

Here are some of the key health benefits of guacamole and sliced vegetables:

1. **Rich in fiber:** Both avocados and vegetables are high in fiber, which helps to promote digestive health and keep you feeling full and satisfied.

2. **Heart-healthy:** The monounsaturated fats in avocados can help to lower cholesterol levels and reduce the risk of heart disease.

3. **Nutrient-dense:** Vegetables are loaded with essential vitamins and minerals, including vitamin C, vitamin A, potassium, and folate.

4. **Antioxidant-rich:** Many vegetables contain antioxidants, which help to protect against cellular damage and may reduce the risk of chronic diseases like cancer and heart disease.

5. **Low in calories:** Guacamole and sliced vegetables are low in calories, making them a great choice for weight management.

6. **Gluten-free and vegan-friendly:** This recipe is naturally gluten-free and vegan-friendly, making it suitable for a wide range of dietary needs.

Incorporating guacamole and sliced vegetables into your diet is a great way to boost your overall health and wellbeing. It's a tasty and satisfying snack that's perfect for any time of day.

Homemade Granola Bars

Granola bars are a convenient and healthy snack option that can be enjoyed at any time of the day. While store-bought granola bars are widely available, they can be expensive and often contain added sugars and preservatives. Making your own homemade granola bars is a simple and affordable way to ensure that you are getting a healthy and nutritious snack.

Homemade granola bars are a nutritious snack that can provide you with energy and important nutrients. They are a great source of fiber, healthy fats, and protein, which can help keep you feeling full and satisfied.

How to Make Homemade Granola Bars

Making homemade granola bars is a simple and straightforward process that requires only a few ingredients. Here's how to make them:

Ingredients:

- 2 cups of rolled oats
- 1 cup of chopped nuts (such as almonds or walnuts)
- 1/2 cup of seeds (such as pumpkin or sunflower seeds)
- 1/2 cup of dried fruit (such as raisins or cranberries)
- 1/4 cup of honey
- 1/4 cup of coconut oil
- 1 teaspoon of vanilla extract
- 1/2 teaspoon of salt

Instructions:

1. Preheat the oven to 350 degrees Fahrenheit.
2. Line a baking dish with parchment paper.
3. In a large bowl, mix together the oats, nuts, seeds, and dried fruit.

4. In a small saucepan, heat the honey, coconut oil, vanilla extract, and salt until the coconut oil is melted.

5. Pour the honey mixture over the oat mixture and stir until well combined.

6. Pour the mixture into the prepared baking dish and press it down firmly with a spatula.

7. Bake for 20-25 minutes or until the edges are golden brown.

8. Allow the granola bars to cool completely before cutting them into bars.

Nutritional benefits of Homemade granola bars

High in Fiber:

Homemade granola bars are high in fiber, which is essential for maintaining a healthy digestive system. The oats and nuts used in the recipe provide a good source of dietary fiber, which helps regulate bowel movements and prevent constipation. The high fiber content in granola bars also helps you feel full for longer, reducing the urge to snack between meals.

Packed with Nutrients:

Homemade granola bars are packed with nutrients that are essential for maintaining a healthy body. The oats and nuts used in the recipe are rich in protein, healthy fats, and vitamins such as vitamin E and B complex. They are also a good source of minerals such as iron, zinc, and magnesium.

Low in Added Sugar:

Most store-bought granola bars are loaded with added sugars, which can lead to weight gain, tooth decay, and other health problems. Making your own granola bars allows you to control the amount of sugar used in the recipe. You can substitute sugar with healthier alternatives like honey or maple syrup, which provide natural sweetness without the harmful effects of refined sugars.

Versatile:

Homemade granola bars are highly versatile and can be customized to suit your taste preferences. You can add a variety of ingredients such as dried fruits, chocolate chips, or seeds to make the bars more interesting and flavorful. You can also adjust the amount of nuts and seeds used in the recipe to increase the protein content.

Conclusion

Incorporating juicing into your diet can be a great way to increase your daily intake of fruits and vegetables, and can provide a number of potential health benefits, including improved digestion, increased energy, and a strengthened immune system. However, it's important to keep in mind that juicing should be used in combination with a balanced diet, rather than as a replacement for whole foods.

For cancer patients specifically, juicing may offer additional benefits, such as increased nutrient absorption and potential cancer-fighting properties. However, it's important to speak with a healthcare professional before incorporating juicing into your cancer treatment plan, as certain fruits and vegetables may interact with medications or negatively impact treatment outcomes.

Ultimately, whether you're a cancer patient or simply looking to improve your overall health, juicing can be a delicious and convenient way to add more nutrients to your diet. By keeping these tips in mind and consulting with a healthcare professional as needed, you can safely and effectively incorporate juicing into your daily routine.